Carnivore Diet

The Most Simple Diet For Meat Lovers To Burn Fat Fast, Get Rid Of Food Allergens, Digestion And Skin Issues

Table of Contents

Introduction

Is the carnivore diet right for you? Does the idea of only eating meat and other animal products sound like something you could do? Better yet, does it sound like something you would want to do? We all know someone who doesn't care much for green leafy things, and if that someone is you, the carnivore diet might be just the ticket. This is the diet for people who hate the word 'diet' and love a nice steak. The "diet" is simple enough - it's all in the name!

The carnivore diet, as you probably know, entails strictly eating animal meat, and nothing else; no plant-based foods, no fruit or vegetables, or any processed carbohydrate foods like cereals, breads, and grains. The carnivore diet is designed to have you totally subsist on fatty meats, especially meats like beef, lamb, goat, venison, or pork. Processed meats like sausage, salami, pepperoni and other deli meats can be eaten, but not if they have any fillers, so reading labels becomes increasingly important. Other meats, like fish, chicken, and other, potentially exotic meats like elk, rabbit, and bison are all on the list, although some of these meats are low fat and will need to be supplemented or cooked in a manner that adds fat. So long as you are not lactose intolerant or suffer from any other similar ailments, dairy items like milk, butter, hard cheeses and heavy whipping cream are also allowed, but some proponents of the carnivore diet eschew these additions, only focusing on the meats.

Remember that this diet is designed to have you consuming fat alongside the meat, and if you are consuming lower fat meats, feel free to increase the fat using lard, ghee (a clarified butter product often used in Indian foods), or duck fat. Season the food with any non-plant derived spices that you desire, so long as you aren't breading them or adding cornstarch for frying. Sodium is highly present in a lot of processed meats but be sure to include sodium in your cooking of other meats to prevent cramping muscles and to keep your electrolytes high.

As far as drinks are concerned, you should consume a large quantity of water. Some hot drinks, such as coffee and tea are also permitted, but only if they are not adulterated with sugar or any other additional carbohydrates. Avoid any hot or cold beverages with any carbs like sodas (diet or otherwise, as the diet drink's sweetness may cause additional cravings), vegetable drinks (like V8), fruit juices, energy drinks (again, even the zero carb ones can cause cravings and make your diet harder to follow). Also, avoid protein supplements (which, considering the amount of protein you will be consuming from the meat will absolutely not be necessary). As mentioned above, some people on the carnivore diet avoid dairy and also don't take vitamin supplements, subsisting entirely on animal protein. Also, it is recommended to drink lots of water, and no vegetables, fruits, pasta, grains, legumes, nuts, seeds or plant-based spices, oils or seasonings.

How does it differ from the Keto Diet?

Unlike the now well-known keto diet, the carnivore diet doesn't just reduce the amount of carbohydrates consumed, it effectively eliminates them. As a polar opposite diet to the vegetarian or vegan diets, the animal protein and fat diet claims that not only can we survive on a meat-only diet, we can thrive on it. Not only that, but some proponents of the diet say that vegetables can actually be detrimental to your health. This flies in the face of all of our previous studies and conventional wisdom concerning our human nutritional needs.

The food pyramid gets notably smaller if you eliminate all carbohydrates, fruits and vegetables from the base, but this diet isn't as crazy as it sounds, and, unlike the keto or paleo diets, this one doesn't require you to count calories, watch your carb intake, or figure out complicated substitution recipes. It is strictly subsisting on meat, organs, and even marrow - if it walks, crawls, swims, or flies, you can eat it!

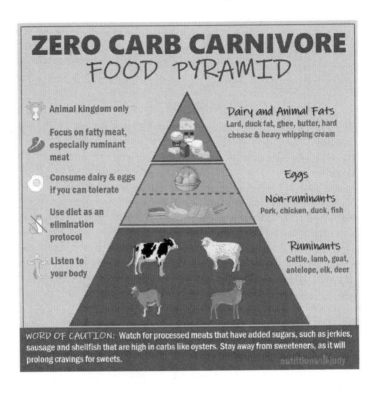

With front facing stereoscopic vision for hunting, and a combination of grinding and tearing teeth (there is a reason why they call those pointy teeth in your head 'canines') – humans are designed to eat meat. But ONLY meat? Read on to see why this diet is not just some new fad, but has real merit. Just because we are all omnivores, it is not just possible to survive on an all-meat diet, we can thrive on it. The diet is technically a zero-carb diet, or all-meat protein diet. Someone following the diet to the letter will only eat meat and drink only water. The diet can also be followed in a less strict way, allowing you to drink coffee and tea. Others choose to include secondary animal products such as dairy and eggs.

Chapter 1: Has Anyone Done This Before?

You may be asking if there's any historical precedent for people living long-term on an all-meat diet, and it's a fair question. Very few cultures have ever tried to live on meat alone. The Inuits are the most well-known group that subsists on an almost exclusive meat and high-fat diet. This isn't by choice, of course, there simply isn't any way to grow anything in the Arctic regions that they inhabit. The fact of the matter is, however, that they not only live, but live well and thrive on their diet. The following sections of this book will discuss not only the health effects, but willfully define the carnivore diet.

What are the claims made about this diet? Proponents of the diet claim that it can help people lose weight, and contrary to popular claims, it can actually improve your cardiovascular health, or increase mental clarity. It is also claimed to alleviate certain autoimmune symptoms, clear up acne and other skin issues and ease depression and anxiety. This diet isn't new, with a recorded historical proponent of the diet being a famous Harvard-trained ethnologist Vilhjalmur Stefansson, who was born in Manitoba in 1879. He spent over a decade exploring the Arctic, nine years of which he lived, and ate, like the Inuit, almost exclusively on meat and fish. He and a colleague agreed, in a funded grant by the American Meat

Packers, to agree to solely subsist on only meat for one year, not in the Arctic, but while living and writing and lecturing in New York. The men lost some weight during the first week of the adjustment period, but maintained a steady weight afterward. Note that the men were not trying to lose weight, so they ate enough meat to maintain their weights. They spent the entire year living entirely on meat and water and claimed that there was no evidence of any loss of physical or mental vigor. There was no evidence that the all-meat diet causes an elevation in blood pressure, nor was there any evidence of vitamin deficiencies.

Remember, that this is not a new diet, rather the opposite. It has gained popularity recently due to its ease and simplicity, as well as the fact that the results for most of the thousands that try this diet speak for themselves.

Chapter 2: Why not ANY Fruits or Vegetables?

The theory is that lectins, gluten and phytic acid found in many plants, rather than being helpful to the system, are actually toxic to humans. Lectins, in particular, have been singled out as seriously detrimental. Lectins, found in seeds, grains, skins, rinds and leaves, protect plants from predators. They have been shown to cause inflammatory reactions like gas, bloating, and more serious health problems. The far more well-known medical complication, celiac disease, has made a significant impact on the way we shop and eat in the past few years, as evidenced by the prolific use of "gluten-free" in packaging and restaurant menus, but what exactly is it, and just how common is the disease?

Celiac disease is a serious condition that causes an immune reaction to eating gluten which harms the small intestine, and in the long term, affects the way your body absorbs nutrients. It affects roughly 1 in 100 people in the world. That means that as many as 2.5 million Americans are undiagnosed and are at risk for long-term health complications from the consumption of gluten. This isn't the same as those who claim sensitivity to gluten, which can cause bloating, gas, discomfort, and can even cause skin conditions similar to eczema at the elbow and knee joints. When people with celiac disease eat gluten, which is a protein found in wheat, rye and barley, their body engages the small intestine with an immune system response. These attacks eventually will damage the villi, small fingerlike projections that line the small intestine. These villi are necessary, as they promote nutrient absorption. The damage keeps the villi from doing their job, which is to absorb nutrients. Celiac disease is genetic, meaning that you get it from your family. Therefore, those with a first-degree relative who is affected, such as a child, parent, or sibling have a higher risk of developing celiac disease. All of these problems are completely avoided by putting yourself on the carnivore diet.

How is this Different from the Paleo Diet?

The diet also differs from the so-called paleo diet for many of the same reasons. The paleo diet, so called because when you are following the paleo diet, you can eat anything we could hunt or gather; things like meats, fish, nuts, leafy greens, regional veggies, and seeds. The meat in the Paleolithic area was exceptionally lean, and our ancestors also ate extremely fibrous local plants alongside their nuts, berries, and other fruits and vegetables. Nothing that was specifically cultivated, grown, or farmed is allowed in the paleo diet, let alone the unpleasant fact that life expectancy during that era was approximately 30 years. Not too great a track record for us to try and emulate. The carnivore diet is certain to do better than that for most of us, but are there any health factors that we should be concerned about before beginning the carnivore diet?

Chapter 3: What are the Risks?

For starters, too much protein has been believed to be a problem for those with kidney disease. In fact, this diet may not be well suited to anyone who has a known problem with their kidneys, as the high protein may cause complications that aren't safe. High-protein diets like the carnivore diet and even the keto diet include foods such as red meat and full-fat dairy products, which some studies show may increase your risk of heart disease. It is possible that a prolonged high-protein diet may worsen kidney function in people that already suffer from kidney disease or complications with their kidneys due to other diseases, like diabetes. These complications are potentially dangerous because your body may have trouble eliminating all the waste products of protein-driven metabolism.

Now, before you feel that I am trying to convince you not to try this diet even if you have pre-existing kidney disease, there is good research that disproves eating protein even above the recommended daily allowance, damages kidney function. The opposite is believed to be able to happen according to some studies, and kidney function might even improve by removing excess glucose from your diet and potentially even improve insulin sensitivity. Large amounts of meat have been linked to causing an increase of uric acid in the blood, which can then crystallize in the joints, causing a painful problem known as gout. In the interest of full disclosure, there is also evidence that links consuming excessive amounts of grilled meat to certain types of cancer. When meat, particularly muscle meat instead of things like organ meat, is cooked at high-temperatures, like pan searing or grilling over an open flame, certain chemicals form. These chemicals include heterocyclic amines, which are mutagenic, meaning that they may cause changes in the DNA, that may increase cancer risk, but this would have to be over an extremely long time, and I recommend that you follow the carnivore diet for 30 days at first to try it out and see how your own body reacts. It would be incredibly unlikely that any long-term effect could be complicated in your system in a 30-day period.

Why Should Anyone Try This Diet?

For the same reasons people try any diet. Losing weight, fewer problems with digestion, clearer thinking, fewer allergens, better fitting clothes, and an easy-to-follow diet that allows you to eat the foods you prefer and enjoy. The high protein and fat consumption can increase testosterone in men and could potentially offer other performance benefits for fitness and when exercising. Although the entire diet may seem to be an extreme method, it actually removes all known allergens that cause health issues as simple as stomach cramps or as complex and troublesome as anaphylactic shock. This diet also eliminates gluten, and, just like the other ketogenic diets, can offer many more benefits in a very short period of time.

Experts claim that even though we are designed to eat meat AND plants, plant-based foods are not strictly necessary in the human diet. What do humans require in order to survive? We need protein, fat, vitamins and minerals in certain specific ranges of amounts. Animal foods, especially meat, can cover those needs, and with some simple guidelines, can fulfill our nutritional needs without plants. This does not mean that we should not eat plant matter at all; it just means that technically it isn't necessary, especially in the short-term.

People who are on the carnivore diet do not suffer from any serious vitamin or mineral deficiencies, even those who are not taking supplements. Red meat contains a large amount of zinc and iron, naturally filling those needs and, as long as you follow the diet and include seafood and dairy into your meal rotation, this will fill your needs for vitamin D. Vitamin C is in short supply, which is why a multivitamin supplement is sometimes recommended with the carnivore diet, but some claim that in the absence of carbohydrates and plant-based foods, your need for vitamin C is greatly reduced. Due to the fact that when on a 'balanced' diet consisting of plant-based foods, carbohydrates and protein, vitamin C is necessary for the formation of collagen and prevention of the disease known as scurvy. None of the experts or persons currently on the diet have reported any problems with even the early symptoms of scurvy, which is a disease resulting from a lack of vitamin C (ascorbic acid). Early symptoms include weakness, feeling tired, and sore arms and legs. Without treatment, decreased red blood cells, gum disease, changes to hair, and bleeding from the skin may occur When consuming a high protein and no carbohydrate diet, especially in the short-term, the large amount of amino acids found in red meat supplement that particular building block in your system.

Experts claim that if you eat different types of meats from the range of proteins available to you, that it's more likely that you will be far more likely to get all of the micronutrients you need. Don't just eat steak and bacon every day. Expand your diet to include fatty fish, organ meats like liver and kidneys, and even bone marrow (roasted or in bone broth). You will find that some of these lesser known cuts of meat actually contain more micronutrients than vegetables!

Chapter 4: So, What CAN I Eat?

As stated above, your meals should consist of animal foods alone. That is as it implies - your food sources can only be meat and the other products provided by animals. When should you eat? Whenever you are hungry and eat until you are sated. Here are some examples of foods that you can and should enjoy on the carnivore diet:

Let's start with the obvious – meat, Steak, roasts, burgers (without the vegetables or bun, of course) generally make up the main food source for those on the diet. It is essential that you eat enough calories, because even if red meat is nutrient dense, it is easy to feel full well before you take in enough calories in a day. Eat fattier cuts of meat to ensure you are taking in enough to keep your energy up. Game meats are generally much leaner than store-bought meats, so meat by-products like lard or dairy fats like butter and ghee should be used to supplement the lack of fat in game. Something that should also be mentioned is marrow, which is a soft, fatty substance found inside bones. You can cook down bones in water or create a stock from meat, bones, and salted water (I share a recipe for the broth later in the book). If available from your butcher, you can get femurs from cattle, have them cut lengthwise to expose the marrow, and roast it in the oven for a decadent high fat and nutrient-filled treat.

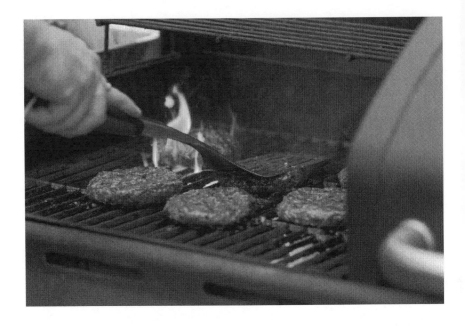

Pork is great, even though most chops and loin are low-fat due to the way pigs are now raised and processed and, speaking of processed, meat products such as sausage and bacon are perfectly fine, so long as they don't use any grains or fillers. Check your labels before you buy sausage or higher processed meats like deli meat, hot dogs, and other meat products. Organ meat, although not as popular as a ribeye steak, should be tried for multiple reasons, as their lack of popularity means generally lower prices, not to mention that they're even more nutrient-rich than some vegetables. Other meats, like any and all seafood, are also fantastic for the diet, not to mention that they allow for quite a bit of variety. Remember that any kind of unprocessed seafood is great, but try to eat higher fat fish, such as salmon or fatty tuna to make sure you are taking in enough calories. If your only experience with poultry is a boneless, skinless chicken breast, you are going to want to expand your poultry repertoire. Again, fattier cuts of poultry, such as the thighs, or the incredibly rich and fat-laden duck and goose meat, are the better choice for you on this diet. Now, let's stretch our definition of meats and animal by-products and talk about eggs.

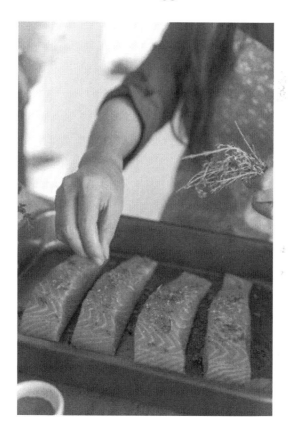

Photo courtesy of Rawpixel on Unsplash

Eggs are a fantastic source of nutrition and protein so

long as you eat the whole egg, and don't separate them. The yolks contain fat and protein in abundance and are a great break from the flavor and texture of meat. Enjoy them as often as you like!

I have spoken about dairy before, but it bears repeating. Although some proponents of the carnivore diet remove milk, butter, cream, yogurt, and cheese from the diet, they do come from animals and are therefore technically available to use. Some people attempting this diet, having learned of it through the keto diet, limit their dairy to allow their bodies to go into ketosis. Other dieters find that they have a negative physical reaction to milk and other dairy products once their bodies have grown used to the new way of eating and getting energy. I recommend that you experiment with dairy items in small doses to see how your body on the diet reacts to them. You may just find that you don't need or miss them at all. I will discuss the differences between the keto and carnivore diets in a later section, but for now just realize that you do have options! The diet can be fun, fulfilling, and fast to show results.

Earlier, I touched on the fact that almost all condiments and seasoning are plant-based, and therefore technically not available to use on the diet, but I cannot see any reason to force yourself to eat only salted meats for the diet. Black pepper and any other calorie-free seasonings should be allowable in the minuscule amounts used to season meat. Avoid any condiments that add calories to your meal, or things like ketchup or barbecue sauces, which are not only made up of plant materials, but also sugar. As you are going to be eating highly flavorful things like fatty rich meats, you may find that you no longer want anything else on your steak but a little salt, pepper, and perhaps a little butter to finish. While seasoning blends are an easy solution, make sure that they do not have any sugar or calories. Again, the purist will just use meat and salt, but that's one of the beauties of this diet. There are levels of this diet and all of them are valid, like vegetarians and vegans.

What Can I Drink?

Moving on to beverages; water is key. Drink your full sixty-four ounces of water daily, keeping yourself hydrated and helping protect your kidneys. Although some carnivore dieters drink strictly water, others have found that drinking coffee or tea without sugar helps boost their day, and even though they're certainly not animal products, you may find that your metabolism increases with the addition of caffeine. Remember, if you are including dairy into your diet, you can certainly adulterate your coffee with milk or cream. Speaking of milk and cream, both of which contain a certain amount of carbohydrates from natural sugars, just what is the difference between the carnivore diet and the keto diet?

How is this Different from those other Diets Again?

The carnivore diet and ketogenic diet both allow the dieter to consume proteins and fats, while simultaneously lowering the intake of carbohydrates. With the keto diet, these carbohydrates are restricted, but they are still able to consume several low carbohydrate vegetables, nuts, and even a small amount of grains, as long as they keep their daily intake of carbohydrates between 5 and as much as 20% of their caloric intake per day.

Chapter 5: Don't I Need Some Carbohydrates?

There is, of course, no way to completely eliminate carbs, as your body actually learns to make them to fuel the activities you need your body to perform. This process is gluconeogenesis. Our bodies need glucose to survive. The "normal" way that we get glucose is through the direct consumption of it in the forms of sugars, simple, and complex carbohydrates which are broken down in the digestive tract and distributed throughout the body. The brain requires energy that comes from glucose, but the body can only store enough glucose to last for less than two hours.

What happens to your body and brain if you only consume meat or if you drastically lower your carbohydrate intake? The process, as stated above, is called gluconeogenesis, which is a pathway used by the body to create glucose from other molecules. This is the process that quite literally prevents us from dying if we've not had any carbohydrates for a few hours. What both the keto diet, so named for the diet's intent to put yourself into a state of ketosis, and the carnivore diet have in common is this process that the body does naturally using some amino acids and triglycerides, abundant in red meat. So, even though the keto and carnivore diets rely on the reduced intake of carbs, calling either of the diets low or no carbs doesn't really describe them on a molecular level. The body will take or make glucose to help keep our brains and bodies in perfect working order. On the carnivore diet, it does not matter if your body goes into or maintains ketosis, but what the heck is ketosis anyway? When your body is low in carbohydrates, your blood sugar levels go down too, thus leading to breaking down the fat to use as energy. Ketoacidosis is a more serious form of ketosis - a dangerous condition for people, particularly diabetics. Ketosis may not be dangerous, as many experts say ketosis itself is not necessarily harmful, but if you have diabetes (type 1 or 2), you could be in serious trouble. As stated before, the carnivore diet isn't dependent upon putting your body into ketosis, so the diet may be a better fit than the keto diet for those millions of people suffering from diabetes, but let's talk about diabetic ketoacidosis so that you know the warning signs. It is a serious complication for diabetics that happens when the body produces high levels of blood acids called ketones.

The condition develops when your body can not produce enough insulin, which can be triggered by a low-carb diet. Insulin allows glucose to enter your cells. Without enough insulin, your body begins to break down fat as fuel, which both diets are relying upon. This process, however, in a diabetic produces a build-up of acids in the bloodstream called ketones, eventually leading to diabetic ketoacidosis if untreated. If you have diabetes or you are at risk of diabetes, learn the warning signs of diabetic ketoacidosis and know when to seek emergency care. Diabetic ketoacidosis symptoms often develop quickly, possibly able to be in full ketoacidosis within 24 hours. You may notice excessive thirst, frequent urination, nausea and vomiting, abdominal pain, weakness or fatigue, shortness of breath, fruity-scented breath, confusion, high blood sugar level (hyperglycemia), or high ketone levels in your urine. Keeping all of this in mind will help both people with and without diabetes follow the diet safely.

Are There Any Long Term Studies On This Diet?

The carnivore diet is very old, but in some ways incredibly new, and there are no metrics on calories, intake amounts, or percentages of total calories. Because the diet has never been formally studied, the only diet information we have are from the people who have taken this on as a lifestyle. Most of the proponents of this diet agree that red meat from beef cattle, bison, and buffalo are the key to optimal performance. Remember that all of your food must be sourced from animals, stay away from anything else and you are sure to succeed. This is the easiest diet to understand and implement. You can eat any animal food products in any combination or amounts you can think of and, if you decide not to pursue the diet strictly, you open up your meal plans to contain, cheese, milk, cream, sour cream and yogurt, all of which would be severely restricted in a keto diet.

I've spoken at great length regarding the safety and health risks of a low or no-carb diet, but let's move forward into the benefits! Some of these may surprise you!

Chapter 6: What Are the Benefits?

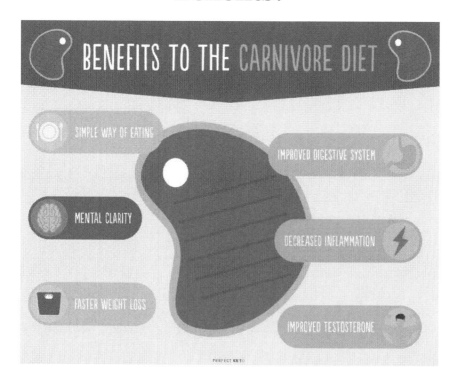

Image courtesy of Perfect Keto

The first benefit seems counter-intuitive, but you are almost guaranteed to lose weight on the carnivore diet.

You read that right. You WILL most likely lose weight on an all-meat diet.

Even with all of that additional fat? Absolutely. Meat dishes, especially those with a high fat content are very rich. Without the bulk of carbohydrates or vegetable matter, your body will become a more efficient machine, keeping your blood sugar low and constant. The process of ketosis that I described above will help your system run as a more efficient muscle-building machine.

After gaining weight due to being idle for a long time because of a knee injury, Andy decided to give the diet a shot for 90 days. As he started the diet, he had a body weight of 214 pounds, body fat percentage of 30.6, and a waist circumference of 35". After 45 days, he tested his body fat and found that it dropped down to 27.6. At the end of the diet, his body weight dropped by 30 pounds, and his body fat dropped to around 24 percent. Also, his shrink circumference had shrunk up to 32". He claimed to have felt perfectly fine during the whole 90 days, and he did not notice any his mood or mental health, as some other people have experienced. He noted that while he did lose 30 pounds, on a low carb diet such as this one, you lose a lot of water weight, so all the weight he lost wasn't pure fat, though he knew his reduction in body fat was notable as he took pictures of himself before and after the diet.

Experts who have gone on the diet found themselves losing body fat, weight, and feeling more clear-minded. Although it may seem strange eating anywhere between two and four pounds of meat every day, it didn't take long to get used to it, to fantastic results! All I ask is that you give the diet a chance to make a fantastic change in your life. A 30-day trial will show you just how effective this diet can be. You will make tremendous strides in the elimination of cravings, removal of toxins, and surprisingly effective weight loss, but the diet must be followed to work. No snacking, binging, or cheat days. It may seem like a lot to ask, but it really will take off the weight if you stick to the plan. If you aren't trying the diet for weight loss, just adjust the amount of meat that you eat to stabilize your body. There are well-known athletes and physical trainers who had to adjust their diets to take in closer to four pounds of meat every day to keep at their peak weight. Even though the diet can naturally put you into ketosis, please remember that that is not the primary goal of the carnivore diet. Ketosis can be a way to rapidly lose weight, and it's just one of the potential side effects of this diet.

What Are Some Other Benefits?

For the male dieter, another possibly surprising effect of the diet is the increase of testosterone. When you undergo a diet high in fat, it has been reported that this may increase your testosterone levels.

Published studies have shown that a high-protein high-fat diet can increase testosterone levels in adults by almost 15%! If you are having any sort of the myriad problems caused by a lack of testosterone or low-T, this diet should do you, and your partner, several favors. But what about the most obvious problem faced by consuming such a large amount of saturated fats? What will this diet do to your heart? As it turns out, not a lot. At least, nothing bad. Regardless of conventional wisdom, there is still no evidential link between fats, saturated or unsaturated, and heart disease. New studies state that you should look at your cholesterol ratio rather than your total cholesterol, which can be calculated by dividing your total cholesterol number by your HDL score. To calculate your cholesterol ratio, divide your total cholesterol number by your HDL cholesterol number so, if your total cholesterol is 200 mg/dL (5.2 mmol/L) and your HDL is 50 mg/dL (1.3 mmol/L), your ratio would be 4-to-1. Higher ratios mean a higher risk of heart disease. These levels and ratio have been shown to actually lower after a month on the diet, but bear in mind that everyone's body is different, and you should always check with your doctor or physician before starting any new diet.

Anything Else?

Further potential benefits are a reduction in the inflammation of your joints. Although there been multiple studies that get cherry-picked by vegetarians that state that a high-fat, high-animal protein diet can cause or increase inflammation, peer-reviewed studies have compared people who ate a high in fat and low in carbohydrate diet with their opposite. The expected results are that the low in fat and high carbohydrates would have less inflammation around their joints, but the study found that the opposite was true.

According to some vegan literature, foods rich in fat cause an inflammation that is just as bad as that caused by smoking cigarettes. However, the reality is that it can actually reduce it. In 2013, a journal called Metabolism conducted a study comparing those who ate a high-fat, low carb diet to those with a low-fat, high-carb diet. While both groups could only eat a certain amount of calories, the study showed that those who ate high-fat were less affected by inflammation after twelve weeks. Therefore, the researchers deduced that eating such a diet may be more favorable to cardiovascular health. This may be due to the fact that several people may have a low-grade intolerance to many of the foods we eat daily. By eliminating all of these plants and carbohydrates from our diet in one fell swoop by starting the carnivore diet, it can remove all of that inflammation quickly. Not to mention the benefits of eating proteins high in gelatin, collagen, and marrow, which have been shown to also lower inflammation and help fix painful or stiff joints, therefore, the carnivore diet will help you find the things that are causing you discomfort quite quickly.

That's not all, though. The carnivore diet has been reported to be great for digestion as well. Christina, who had terrible constipation her whole life, decided to try the diet for a week, and was initially worried that it would actually worsen it. However, by the second day, she already felt great, as her bloating was gone. She did have loose stools for two days out of the first week, but she suspected that this was caused by the ghee she was using, and once she stopped consuming it, claimed that she never had better bowel movements in her entire life.

All around, I felt amazing the first week, especially with my digestion. I was wrong to worry about becoming constipated because, if anything, the opposite happened. There were about two days when I had loose stools, but that evened out. I'm still not sure if that was because of the ghee I was using (I do react to ghee when I use too much of it), or because my fat:protein ratio was too high. I stopped using ghee and ate slightly less fat, and things evened out. After that, I had never had better bowel movements in my life! That obviously put me in a good mood.

After you have completed your 30-day trial of the diet, if you decide not to carry on with it, I advise that you very slowly reintroduce things such as grains, pasta, and other carbohydrates one at a time, giving each of them a few meals to see how your newly trained digestive tract reacts to each one. Adding them in one meal at a time, you will be able to find what 'normal' fruits, vegetables and carbohydrates to avoid in the future.

Another thing that flies in the face of current dietary beliefs, you can find that you have fewer gastrointestinal issues. In a world that has preached the extreme benefits of fiber, and its necessity for 'moving the mail' as it were, these beliefs could be entirely wrong. People with unknown sensitivities to gluten, lectins, and the phytic acid in fruits, vegetables, grains, nuts, and seeds may find that these foods contribute to inflammation and auto-immune disorders. Of course, this is simply an opinion rather than a proven reason. The fact is that so many people on the carnivore diet have fewer digestive problems, less gas, and even reduced Irritable Bowel Syndrome means that there must be some merit to the claims. Grains, nuts, and seeds may find that these foods contribute to inflammation and auto-immune disorders.

Chapter 7: What Is Being On the Diet Like?

With all low or no carbohydrate diets, there's an adjustment period where you will likely feel tired and have minor mood swings as your body adjusts to the new diet and how to keep you going. This is often referred to as the 'Keto flu' because the body aches, mild fevers, and lethargy are all common symptoms but, if you give it a week or so to break-in, you should feel better, sharper and more focused. After this adjustment period, consistently in ketosis or not, you should have a mental clarity to rival any other time in your life. And finally, one of the most fantastic benefits of this diet is its pure simplicity. If carb-counting, calorie checklists, and number coded meals have always been your downfall, welcome to the easiest diet you will ever try.

Once you decide whether you are going to go a pure carnivore diet or allow yourself dairy (always start with small amounts and work your way up), the diet is completely self-explanatory. While meat can be expensive, if it is the only thing you are buying, then you will find your overall purchase cost should be lower. Quality meats may seem pricey when viewed separately, but realizing it to be your total cost should allow you to splurge and get new and exciting cuts or focus on that beautiful ribeye and treat yourself, every meal! Your diet is literally eating animal foods when you are hungry and eating until you are full. That's it. That's the entire diet. No scales. No color codes. No set meal times or snacks or cardboard-tasting carob covered bars masquerading as a full meal. Eat meat.

As a matter of fact, people on the diet find that they're hungry less often because fatty meats are naturally more filling, but the question most asked is "is the diet safe?" The short answer is, in the short-term, yes. Could there be health risks should you change to this diet in the long-term? The short answer is we don't know. It has proven to be an efficient way to move your body into burning fat as energy instead of carbohydrates. We know scientifically that meat isn't to blame for heart disease, and there are indigenous groups of people who live their entire lives consuming only meat and fat, but that doesn't mean that it's a one-size-fits-all diet if you decide to continue it as a lifestyle choice. The Inuit people aside, there have been no studies of this diet and its effects in the long-term. One thing that HAS been studied is that red meat makes it through your intestinal tract just fine. There's an urban myth that red meat gets impacted in your gastrointestinal tract if you eat too much of it, and it's simply not true. It may be that on the carnivore diet your bowel movements will be notably smaller than perhaps you are used to, but that is simply because you will no longer be taking in roughage, vegetables, or bulky bread products.

How Long Should I Try This Diet?

Enough speculation about the diet, let's see how you should try it out yourself!

It is strongly recommended that the best way to try out the diet is to do a 30-day version. Choose your start day, go shopping for it, move or hide all of the rest of your staple items to avoid temptation, and stock out your fridge with a few days' worth of meat. If you have a normal Monday through to Friday job, make your start day Saturday, so that you can be home and make your first few meals. This will keep you from being tempted by eating out of the house for the first few days of your diet.

For most people who want to try start eating a meat-only diet, then this one-month challenge is a good way to start. You should use the time to see if you feel better after the initial week or so of adjustment. Take care to notice if you are feeling more energetic, less inflammation, fewer aches and pains, better sleep, and clearer skin. Other health benefits should be easier and less subjective, such as weight loss, less time feeling hungry, better blood sugar results for diabetics, and thyroid levels. Diabetics should also have their A1C checked before and after participating in the diet for 30 days to make sure you are staying healthy and controlling your blood sugar long-term. Also, consider taking before and after pictures, keeping a health diary, and/or tracking these lab results, which will then help you know if this is the diet plan for you or not.

Chapter 8: The Diet

Remember, as always, that diet is as its name suggests is an all-meat and animal products diet. Also, take note that you are going to have to decide whether you will be supplementing your diet with a small number and amount of dairy products. Some choose to do this to ease into the diet or to add in a little variety, as well as some vitamin D. As before, I mentioned that some people take vitamin supplements, so feel free to adjust these few things to your own diet. We know that every person's body is different and will react to the diet in their own way, so please make informed decisions when it comes to your own health and safety. Here is a condensed list of allowable foods on the diet.

Type of Protein	Example Foods
Red Meat	Beef, pork, lamb, wild game, duck, geese, or other wild fowl
White Meat	Chicken, turkey, fish, seafood
Organ Meat	Liver, kidneys, tongue, bone marrow, heart, brain
Eggs	Chicken eggs, goose eggs, duck eggs
Dairy	Heavy cream, whole milk, cheese, butter, ghee

Remember that although meats and dairy are packed with protein, make sure that you eat enough to feel full. Do not just eat lean meats and low-fat options, or you can reduce your caloric intake down to dangerous levels. The natural saturated and unsaturated animal fat on the meat provide necessary daily nutritional needs for your body. Not just the need to keep your calories up to a safe level, but along with the fats and protein, there are necessary vitamins, minerals and amino acids in the meat, not to mention the fact that fat makes food taste better! As you won't be eating any plant matter or plant-based proteins like soy beans, it is necessary to eat until you feel full. As the diet goes on, after your adjustment period, your appetite will likely change. You should not leave any meal until you feel sated, as you will need to eat to your personal needs. Whether you exercise heavily or have a more sedentary lifestyle, eat until you are full. It is approximated that you will need to eat an average of two pounds of meat daily, unless you have a physically demanding job or work out heavily.

When Should I Eat?

When should you eat? When you feel hungry is the basic answer, but it's not the only one. Eating three meals a day is perfectly acceptable; some people feel better having just one or two meals a day. Or if you like, you can stretch out your caloric intake to five or six smaller portions a day. Some even find that intermittent fasting works for them. Intermittent fasting (IF) is an eating pattern that cycles between periods of fasting and eating. It's currently quite popular and has several methods in order to keep your energy up and can be used in this diet. In fact, because it restricts the same things that are restricted here, such as high carbohydrate meals, or detrimental snacking on junk food, it can pair with the carnivore diet to achieve faster results (you will find a link in bonus section to get a copy of a **free e-book about Intermittent Fasting**). Note that this is only for those who are able to do so, due to their daily schedule or by closely monitoring the results and listening to your body's needs, and please remember that no particular method is a one-size-fits-all and that it is optional. With the high caloric and protein rich diet, some people do find themselves less hungry and can easily employ one of the popular methods of IF. As this is a potentially useful method to add in more health benefits, here are listed the most popular variants of IF:

The 16/8 method: Also known as Leangains, this method involves skipping breakfast and restricting your daily eating period to 8 hours, such as 12–8 p.m. This simple method by its nature has you fasting for 16 hours in between.

TIME-RESTRICTED FEEDING
16:8

FAST
16 Hours

EAT
8 Hours

Image courtesy of Metabolic Meals

The 5:2 diet: With this method, you only consume 500–600 calories on 2 non-consecutive days of the week, but eat normally the other 5 days. Like the Eat-Stop-Eat method, take care not to fast on consecutive days (like the weekend) as this could cause you too serious a drop in caloric intake. This method also has the added difficulty of counting calories, which adds some complexity to our simple carnivore diet.

Eat-Stop-Eat: This involves fasting for 24 hours and should only be done once or twice a week, or you could find yourself losing too much energy and actually be starving your body, slowing your metabolism. The easiest example is simply not eating from dinner one day until your dinner on the next day.

Any of these methods can be easily added to the carnivore diet, and only you can know if any of them are right for you. Please do NOT employ any of these methods until after your adjustment period, as your body needs time to adjust to this new way of eating and drinking.

Stay Hydrated!

Speaking of drinking, I cannot emphasize enough the necessity of keeping yourself hydrated with plenty of water. Depending upon how strict you want to be on the diet, I recommend you try and drink only water for your 30-day trial. It can be any type of non-flavored water, such as tap, sparkling, or filtered water. You may need to add a little salt to your water to avoid muscle cramps and other issues. Tea and coffee are not technically allowed (as they both have their flavors derived from plant matter), but as long as you only add cream, milk, or 'bulletproof' your coffee with butter, you can have your precious caffeine without any adverse effects to the diet.

Chapter 9: What CAN I Eat And Where Do I Get It?

As I have stated before, the diet is as simple as it can get. Only animal-derived protein is allowed, but how do you cook it? On this diet, you can cook any of your proteins to your desired doneness. Although restaurants and chefs agree that you should not cook a good piece of beef to anything past medium rare to truly enjoy the flavor and tenderness of a good cut of steak, you are free to cook your proteins to any level of doneness you wish. The mineral, proteins, vitamins, and amino acids do not reduce any significant amount unless you cook the steak beyond well done. Some game meats are recommended to only cook them to medium rare as well, but that again is up to your personal preference.

Some meats, namely most farmed poultry such as chicken and turkey, should be cooked more fully to make sure that they are safe to eat. Pork is another example that has a safe internal temperature of 145 degrees Fahrenheit, for health reasons. Fish and other seafood can be consumed from raw to cooked completely dry. Experiment! Go out for sushi or fresh oysters, but naturally, you will need to get it without the rice or other vegetable-derived accouterments.

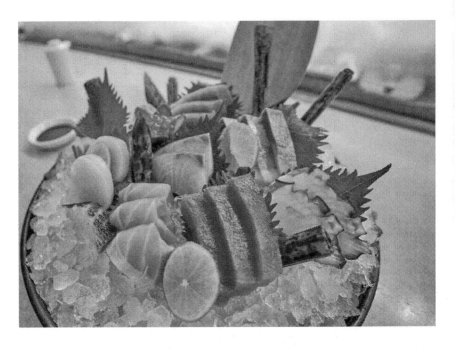

Image courtesy of Jongsun Lee on Unsplash

If you wish to experiment at home with these sorts of things, it's important that you get the freshest seafood you can find and follow these simple rules for selecting and preparation of raw fish. First and foremost, you need to avoid albacore tuna and King mackerel, as they contain high levels of mercury. Lower mercury options include salmon and freshwater trout. Mercury is a heavy metal toxin that can build up in the blood and cause neurological problems, impairing memory and fine motor skills. Average adults won't get mercury poisoning from an occasional sushi dinner as that would require eating large amounts of high-mercury fish, but consuming less mercury is always better than consuming more. Pregnant women and adults 65 and older, or people with a weakened immune system, are particularly sensitive to mercury's effects so eating any raw fish should be off limits to these groups. You should also make sure that you are buying your fish from a fishmonger you trust.

Buy your meats from a local butcher shop if you have one, as it is a great place to take your time and ask questions about different kinds and cuts of meat. Most proponents of the diet claim that you should focus on grass-fed and grass-finished beef cuts. Although more expensive than conventional cuts, the experts say the quality of the meat matters. You can also often find excellent deals on organ meat and wonderful advice on how to best prepare it from your local butcher.

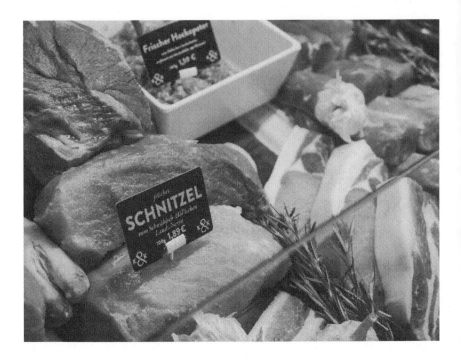

Your local grocery is where most people get their meats, and that's perfectly acceptable. Although it's always best to get the freshest meats available, grocery stores often have some other more frugal options and you will find that every Wednesday the specials change! Speaking for a moment on grocery meat, some people complain that all grocery meat tastes the same due to the additional solutions that are added to lengthen shelf life. This is because the vast majority of the beef sold in grocery stores is aged instead of dry-aged. Wet-aging consists of vacuum packing larger primal or sub-primal cuts in plastic and letting it age in a refrigerator. The meat is packed in its own juices, allowing its natural enzymes to break down connective tissues but without the fluid loss or mold growth of dry aging.

My grandfather told me that all meat tastes like liver these days because of the wet-aging method. This simply would not do! If you have ever had a dry-aged steak in a steakhouse, here is a simple method to get close to that taste and texture at home. A simple trick once you get home with your steaks (I especially like this method for T-bone steaks and ribeyes), is to take them out of the package and wrap them in paper towels before you place them into your refrigerator, on a plate or tray. You will almost immediately see a pink liquid staining the paper towels. Leave them overnight, unwrap them, and then rewrap them in fresh paper towels in the morning, and repeat this again the next morning. This method, in just three or four days, will render the steaks more flavorful, and will allow the fat of the meat to make the steak juicy, instead of the solution they've been prepared within the aging process that is so prevalent in our current grocery stores.

Other Sources for Meat and Dairy

One of the other sources for your meat and animal products like fresh cream, whole milk, and cheese is your local farmer's market. You will have the opportunity to talk to the farmer about their meats and methods they employ, often getting meat and dairy products fresher than any store, although you will be often paying a premium. Remember though, as you are ONLY subsisting on meat, it's alright to splurge on a particularly nice cut. You may even find that even though meat can be quite expensive, you will still be spending less at the store because you are cutting out every other item that is normally on your list. No vegetables, fruits, sodas, chips, or anything else; just meat.

Going further, how you cook your meat will be extremely important to you to keep the diet fun, easy, and interesting. This is why, even though the diet is supposed to be free of any vegetables, herbs, or plant derived spices, I can recommend if you find yourself growing tired of the same flavor profile each meal, there is little harm in using any of the no calorie spice blends. I, of course, recommend that you try with just simple salt and allow for the meat to shine through, but I also understand that people can grow tired of the same thing day in, day out. Seasoning aside, I can also recommend a lot of different gear for getting the most out of your meat.

Chapter 10: What Else Will I Need?

Everything starts with a good cutting board. Before it ever touches a pan, you will be cutting and trimming your meats. Do not over-trim the fat from your meats, as you need those extra calories and the nutrients in the fat. Preparing them on the counter can potentially damage both your counters and contaminate your meat. I prefer a butcher's block, both for sturdiness and simplicity to clean. If you do use a smaller, silicon or self-healing plastic board, an easy trick to keep it from moving or sliding around as you cut, put a damp kitchen towel on the counter first to lock the board in place and, speaking of the cutting, you will want a quality knife that can keep an edge. Familiarize yourself with the different types of blades and which one helps you trim and cut your meats for you. A chef's knife set will contain all of the types of blades you will need, but if you are going to invest in any sort of quality brand blade, make sure you keep it sharp and let the blade do the work for you.

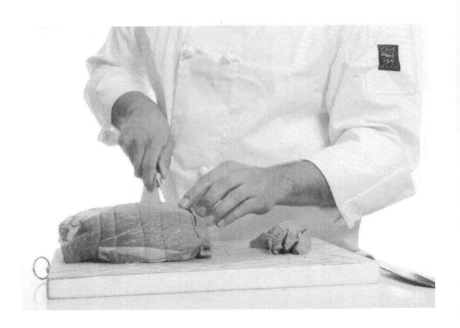

Image courtesy of Marvin Tolentino on Unsplash

You may have seen chefs on television using a steel rod before they cut. That particular tool, simply called a 'steel,' doesn't actually sharpen the blade but, instead, lines up the already-sharpened edge into a single line, making the blade cut through almost anything with ease. Make sure you also have steak knives! Your staple food is going to be red meat steaks, marbled and tender, certainly, but you will still need to get the thing down to bite sized pieces at the table. Finally, how are you going to be preparing these meals? I suggest cast iron, either in skillet or grill pan form. You will find that cast iron, once properly seasoned, will allow your steaks to get a good sear on the outside and remain juicy and succulent inside. The grill pan will sear those marks into the meat we all like to see, but it also suspends the steaks above their own fat, allowing for a slightly drier finish.

If the rest of your meals are lower fat, you may want to skip the use of a grill pan as you need to be consuming that fat for energy. Some people prefer the enamel coated cast iron for more of a non-stick surface, and they are certainly preferred over the Teflon-coated pans. Any and all of these types of pans can be used, although you will have a hard time with eggs in the uncoated cast iron, just like you won't get as good a sear or finish on a steak in a Teflon coated pan. It's all up to you, but I want to make sure you get the best possible results with your food.

It is also highly recommended that you get a meat thermometer and familiarize yourself with how it works and reading it properly. As you will be changing your diet so dramatically, it becomes more important than ever to measure the temperatures of your meats accurately. You should always insert the thermometer into the thickest part of the meat, and make sure that you are familiar with the proper safe temperatures for your meals. Always pull your meats off of the heat a few degrees lower than the recommended temperature as there is always a certain amount of carry-over cooking that happens between the grill and the plate. Later in the book, I'll talk about cooking times, or more correctly, the cooking temperatures, for all of the different meats and proteins to get more consistent results, but, for now, just make sure you are using the best tools you can so that you get the best results for your meals.

A Sample Day on the Carnivore Diet

The following is an example of healthy nourishment for a day to get a wide variety of nutrition from a diet involving only animal products:

Breakfast

Black coffee (if you decide to avoid the 'only water' rule). You can have it black, or with cream (not creamer!), or whole milk

Scrambled eggs and bacon

Lunch

Ribeye steak, or the equivalent amount of beef or chicken liver, seasoned with salt and pepper

Snack

1 cup bone broth, OR a few slices of a hard cheese like Colby, cheddar, Emmental, or Manchego

Dinner

Hamburger patty OR salmon fillet

Make sure that each of your animal derived foods is of the highest quality that you can comfortably afford. Grass-fed beef is better than typical grocery meats for flavor and consistency. It's not a requirement, of course, but you will likely find better cuts mean better meals and potentially better health.

Safe Temperatures for Prepared Meats

Use this chart from Foodsafety.gov (the American Federal Food Safety site) and a food thermometer to ensure that meat, poultry, seafood, and other cooked foods reach a safe minimum internal temperature.

Remember, it's important to know if a meat is safe to eat, and this can be hard to tell, as some uncured red meats, such a pork can be pink even when it has reached a safe temperature.

As you take the meat off the grill, or wherever you are cooking it from, let it rest for a little while, as this helps get rid of harmful germs.

Do not ignore resting time, as the fibers in the meat need a little time to reabsorb the liquids that were recently so active. If you cut into a steak the moment you remove it from the heat, you will find the meat dry and get a plate full of pink protein liquid instead of that juicy steak we all want.

Category	Food	Temperature (°F)	Rest Time
Ground Meat & Meat Mixtures	Beef, pork, veal, lamb	160	None
	Turkey, chicken	165	None
Fresh Beef, Veal, Lamb	Steaks, roasts, chops	145	3 minutes
Poultry	Chicken & turkey, whole	165	None
	Poultry breasts, roasts	165	None
	Poultry thighs, legs, wings	165	None
	Duck & goose	165	None
	Stuffing (cooked alone or in bird)	165	None
Pork and Ham	Fresh pork	145	3 minutes
	Fresh ham (raw)	145	3 minutes
	Precooked ham (to reheat)	140	None

Eggs & Egg Dishes	Eggs	Cook until yolk and white are firm.	None
	Egg dishes	160	None
Seafood	Fin Fish	145 or cook until flesh is opaque and separates easily with a fork.	None
	Shrimp, lobster, and crabs	Cook until flesh is pearly and opaque.	None
Seafood	Clams, oysters, and mussels	Cook until shells open during cooking.	None
	Scallops	Cook until flesh is milky white or opaque and firm.	None

Recipes and Tricks of the Trade

Also, with a little creativity, you can enjoy many of the dishes you crave with a few simple adjustments. When people think of the diet, they imagine a large chunk of charred meat, eaten without any sauce or seasonings. Admittedly, if you are going to be following the diet to the letter, this is generally true, but adding the dairy into the meal plan and, in addition, allowing zero calorie versions of seasonings, you can create dishes that are surprising in their flavor and appearance. For example, a relatively new version of the old kitchen standby device, the pressure cooker, has been updated and simplified. Using one of these, such as the Instant Pot, can allow for some particularly tasty innovations.

Although this book is more about the diet than recipes, I feel that the following recipe is an interesting enough use of the allowable ingredients to make something quite different than you might expect with an all-meat meal plan. Admittedly, this is for the people who are not following the strictest interpretation of the carnivore diet, but this is to show that the diet does not have to be just a slab of meat on a plate. Full disclosure, it does add plant matter back into your diet with the garlic, chopped dill, and onion powders. If you are concerned that these things may be too much, omit them or perhaps use this dish as a way to ease yourself back out of the diet. There is also the very real possibility that the plant matter, as small an amount as it is, could be one of the problem items with your metabolism. Referred to as 'crack chicken' or 'King Ranch' chicken, the following will supply you with leftovers for several meals or a good shared dish with friends who aren't joining you on your new diet. It can help promote the diet with your friends and family who are hard to convert!

"Crack" or King Ranch Chicken

Ingredients

2-4 slices bacon chopped into lardon, or small pieces

2-3 lbs boneless, skinless chicken breasts (don't worry, you are adding fat with the cream cheese and heavy cream)

1 8-ounce block of cream cheese

Splash of vinegar for bite (optional)

1 cup heavy cream

½ cup water

1½ teaspoons garlic powder

1 tablespoon onion powder

1 teaspoon crushed red pepper flakes

1 teaspoon dried dill

¼ teaspoon salt

¼ teaspoon black pepper

½ cup shredded cheddar

Instructions

Turn your pressure cooker on, and press "Sauté," then wait a few minutes for the pot to heat up. Add the chopped bacon and cook until crispy. Transfer the bacon to a plate and set aside. Press "Cancel" on the machine to stop sautéing. Add the chicken, cream cheese, water, vinegar (if you are using it), garlic powder, onion powder, crushed red pepper flakes, dill, salt, and black pepper to the pot. Turn the pot on Manual, High Pressure for 20 minutes and then do a quick release. These instructions are for the Instant Pot, but the other versions of the same type of device all use similar buttons. This dish can also be prepared in a crock pot by setting it and letting it go on low for 6 hours or until the chicken can be easily pulled apart with two forks, as described in the next step. Use tongs to transfer the chicken to a large plate, shred it with 2 forks, and return it back to the pot. Stir in the cheddar cheese or serve the chicken mixture and top it with some of the shredded cheddar and a sprinkling of crispy bacon.

This dish is more keto than carnivore, but it does show that the diet can be interesting and more palatable than the repeated meal of salted steak or fish. If you are doing this diet to help you eliminate possible allergens, you may wish to skip this dish entirely as it does reintroduce more than one plant-based seasoning at once.

Bone Broth

Some other preparations can be made in advance for a quick pick-me-up or snack, such as the before-mentioned bone broth. It also takes quite a long time to simmer and become the rich and satisfying addition to your diet that it can be. Here is a detailed recipe for it, using either the carcass from roasted chickens, or beef bones, available from your local butcher or most larger grocery stores.

Bone Broth Ingredients

2 pounds (or more) of bones, roasted

2 chicken feet per gallon extra gelatin (optional but highly recommended)

1 gallon of water

2 tablespoons apple cider vinegar (can be avoided, but it does help the bones release their nutrients)

Optional items per gallon: 1 tablespoon or more of sea salt, 1 teaspoon peppercorns, and additional herbs or spices to taste. You will need a large stock pot to cook the broth in and a fine mesh strainer for when it is done.

The first step in preparing to make a bone broth is to gather high quality bones. You can find them from sources listed above or save them when you cook, especially if you roast whole chickens. The entire remaining carcass with its bones and additional small amounts of meat that cling to the bones make a perfect start for making the broth. These carcasses can be saved and frozen or used immediately. If you're making a large amount of broth to keep available for snack times or to substitute a low calorie meal, you may want to freeze a few of them until you have enough for at least a gallon of water. Broths are especially good if you are going to be using the previously mentioned intermittent fasting plans, and you will find them to be particularly well suited for the 5-2 method.

It is best to use approximately 2 pounds of bones per gallon of water, which is approximately two or three full carcasses, so use only a half-gallon of water if you're making the broth immediately after carving up your chicken. Chicken feet are usually available from your local butcher and in some grocery stores. If you are lucky enough to have a carnitaria (or Mexican butcher shop/grocery), or an Asian market, you will find them more likely to have chicken feet available. The chicken feet are optional, but they have an enormous amount of collagen and gelatin in them and really make the broth have a better, richer texture.

If you are using raw bones, especially beef bones, it improves flavor to roast them in the oven first. Simply place them in a roasting pan and roast for 30 minutes at 350°F.

Almost all recipes online and written in books use carrots, onions, and celery as well as other plant matter to add flavor to the broth. You will also find that all of the commercially available broths are all done the same way, making it essential that you make your own. After roasting your bones, place the bones in a large stock pot (you will want to have a 5-gallon pot to allow enough room for the bones and water. Pour cool water over the bones before you add some vinegar to the mix. Then, allow it to sit for 20 minutes to half an hour in the cold water. The acidity of the vinegar will allow the nutrients in the bones to be more available. Add any salt, pepper, and spices that you like. Then, boil the broth, and once it is boiling aggressively, let it simmer, until it's done. This is where you will have to set it and forget it, as the extremely long simmering time seem intimidating, but they are necessary to get all of the flavor and nutrients out of the bones. Beef broth should simmer for 48 hours, while chicken or any other poultry should cook for no shorter than 24 hours.

Fish bones can also be used with the same methods and weight ratios, and only need to simmer for eight hours. During the first few hours of simmering, you will need to remove the impurities that float to the surface. There will be less of it than if you had the stock vegetables in your broth, but there will be a frothy/foamy layer that forms on top, and it can be easily scooped off with a big spoon. Throw this foam away. You should check it every 20 minutes or so for the first 2 hours to remove this. It is believed that grass fed or free range, grain-fed poultry give off less foam, but just be sure to scoop it off and discard it.

After the admittedly long simmer times, you should remove the broth from the heat and allow it to cool slightly. Using a fine mesh strainer, pour the broth into storage containers, making sure to allow the strainer to remove all of the bits of bone, meat, and remaining seasonings such as the peppercorns. You can keep the containers in the refrigerator for five to seven days or freeze your leftover broth. I recommend that you drink at least one cup per person per day as a health boost, especially in the winter. One of the better quick uses of the broth is to heat eight to sixteen ounces with a little salt to add flavor and whisk in an egg until the egg is cooked, making a soup with a similar texture to egg drop soup.

The broth can help you get through the 'Keto flu' faster too, as it is extremely easy to digest so the body's reaction to the change of diet can be lessened. If you find yourself actually ill during the diet, or in cases of stomach bugs or vomiting, bone broth often calms the stomach very quickly and can help shorten the duration of the illness. This broth should become a staple in your household, regardless of how long you'll be on the carnivore diet

Beef Liver

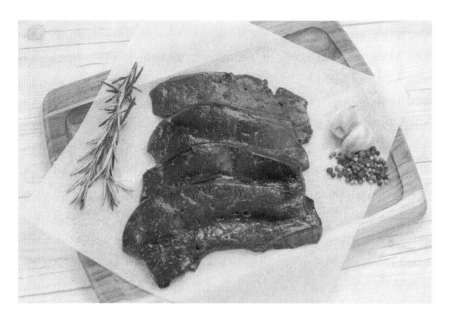

Finally, I will leave you with a recipe for that tricky organ meat, the beef liver. You will likely know the basics for cooking your favorite cuts of beef, and the secret method you have for cooking your perfect roast chicken, but most of us are not used to preparing liver, gizzards, heart, or tongue. This diet is the perfect time to expand your palate!

Many people consider liver to be the most pleasant organ meat. Although it is safe to eat the liver of most food-producing animals, one rule of thumb is this: the younger it is, the better it will taste. Also, whether young or old, liver with will have a musky, metallic taste, and that's why you will often be told to put it in flour before frying it.

As our diet doesn't allow us any flour (or any flour substitute), this recipe is designed to avoid all of that and still make it tasty and crispy outside. Rinse your liver in a colander under cold, running water. It is important to really clean the liver by trimming off all the visible fat, veins and membranes with a paring knife. The veins can be lifted with the tip of a knife; cut them into strips, put them in a bowl of milk and leave it for around half an hour. This will allow all traces of blood and impurities to disappear. Then, remove the strips and rinse the milk off. Finally, dry them off with paper towels.

Heat a scant amount of high-heat, non-plant derived cooking oil (I recommend bacon grease or lard) in a sauté pan over a high heat for about four or five minutes. The oil may start to smoke, but let it get to that point. Season the liver strips on both sides to taste and lower them in the hot oil. Sauté the liver until it's dark, golden brown on the outside, or for about two minutes total. You must keep the strips of liver in motion in order to keep it from burning and allow it to cook evenly. The inside of the liver should be slightly pink for the best taste and texture. Remove the liver from the pan and place it on a plate and serve it immediately. Although liver is usually prepared with onions, we are avoiding all plant matter, so they're definitely out.

Chapter 10: Common Mistakes

By now, you should have realized that this diet isn't as crazy as it first sounds, but there are still additional factors to consider before going on this diet, at least for the long- term. Here are some common mistakes people make when starting this diet:

First and foremost, eating too little food is a common problem. You need to eat until you are full, because even if your primary goal is weight loss, excessive weight loss too quickly can lead to further complications, and actually slow the process later. Another problem common with this diet is not drinking enough water. You shouldn't just drink to quench your immediate thirst, but I recommend that in order to better digest your food and stay hydrated, drink the recommended 64 ounces of water per day or more. Not adding salt to your food is also dangerous and failing to add enough salt to your diet can cause you to have muscle cramps, as well as causing the same symptoms of the so-called Keto flu.

The next, and more obvious common mistake is actually breaking the diet, thinking that you can eat a moderate all-meat diet while allowing yourself to consume even a small amount of added fruits, vegetables, and other types of carbs. Breaking the diet will nullify any good effects, especially in the first 30 days, and, finally, almost the other end of the spectrum of the person who breaks the diet with additional foods. You should not avoid consuming fatty meats. Again, I know that it sounds counter-intuitive, but you need the good cholesterol in the well-marbled and otherwise fattier meats, even if it seems that eating less fat will help you lose weight. Practically speaking, you would have to eat a lot more to reach a safe level of calories to sustain you. Avoiding the fattier meats may also prevent you from entering into ketosis, which, although not the primary goal of this diet, is something many people who go on very low or zero-carb diets are attempting to reach.

There are other concerns as well, both environmentally (if everyone shifted to an all- meat diet, we would rather quickly run out of edible animal protein) and physically. One of the most common questions is if you completely eliminate vegetables and other things high in fiber, is constipation a problem? I touched on this earlier, but it bears repeating that most of the reports by proponents of the diet state that not only is it not a problem, but they find that they're passing smaller stools without the bulk of the usual vegetation and fiber.

Conclusion

In conclusion, this diet has incredibly quick, positive results and very few negatives. Even if you only attempt our 30-day challenge, I am sure that you will be pleased and pleasantly surprised with the results. The proponents of this diet claim dramatic results are just a few weeks away, and the vast variety of fish, fowl, game, pork, poultry, and good old beef should allow you to put a new and interesting meal on your plate every single day! Feel free to experiment with different meats and find a new favorite.

The carnivore diet may not be a one-size-fits-all diet, as it is extremely restrictive, but that is one of the great beauties of the diet; its simplicity. When you adjust your diet as drastically as the carnivore diet, it can be difficult at first. I urge you to stick with it and watch the pounds melt away. If you suffer from allergies, stiffness or aches in your joints, inflammation, bloating, or other gastrointestinal issues, you may seriously find relief in the carnivore diet.

If you decide to end the diet, be sure to give yourself another week to slowly reintroduce vegetables, fruits, and grains and, if possible, reintroduce them one at a time, so that you can really learn how your body reacts to each one. You can effectively find out foods to avoid in just a few weeks of coming off of the diet. As always, when making a significant change to your diet, speak with a dietician or your primary care physician before trying it, but I am sure you'll see incredible results in a very short time. Even if you do not stay on the diet long, the carnivore diet can be a jumping off point to a happier and healthier you!

Finally, if you found this book useful in any way, a review on Amazon is always appreciated!

Free Bonus

Go to link http://bit.ly/cdietbonus and you will get **Free E-Book** about **Intermittent Fasting** to **accelerate** your journey towards **optimum health** and **weight** from today

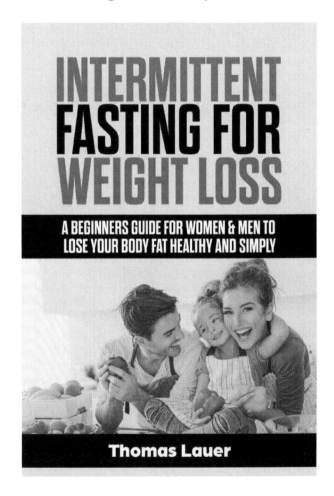

Download the Audio Book Version of This Book for FREE

If you love listening to audio books on-the-go, I have great news for you. You can download the audio book version of this book for **FREE** just by signing up for a **FREE** 30-day audible trial! See below for more details!

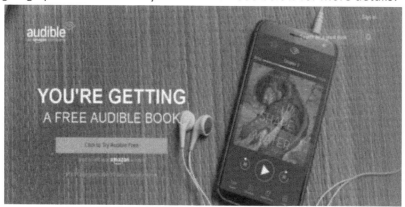

Audible **FREE** 30 day Trial Benefits

- **3 x FREE audible titles** (this book + 2 Audible Originals)
- Listen **anywhere** with the Audible app across multiple devices
- Cancel anytime and **keep all your audiobooks**
- After trial **3 x FREE audible titles** each month
- Choose from Audible's **200,000 +** Titles
- Roll over any unused credits for **up to 5 months**
- Make **easy, no-hassle exchange** of any audiobook you don't love
- **Exclusive** audio-guided wellness programs

Go to the links below to get started!

For Audible US: https://adbl.co/2U2PWKz

For Audible UK: https://adbl.co/2Ommn1p

For Audible FR: http://bit.ly/2Yh2Ofn

For Audible DE: https://adbl.co/2ulv6Yw

47480268R00045